FIT & FAB FOREVER IN 90 DAYS

Weight Management
Tips, Tricks & Secrets Every Professional Woman Over 40 Can Start TODAY!

BY JENI BENNETT

Copyright Information

Credits

Cover design by pro_graphics360

Author photograph by Celine Tiley

Book formatting by thebookformat

Limits of Liability / Disclaimer of Warranty

The Author and publisher of this book

Although the author and publisher have made every effort to ensure that the information in this book was correct at time of printing. The author and publisher do not assume and hereby disclaim any liability to any party for any loss, damage, or disruption caused by errors or omissions, whether such errors or omissions result from negligence, accident, or any other cause.

This book is not intended as a substitute for the medical advice of physicians / doctor. The reader should regularly consult a physician or doctor in matters relating to his/her health and particularly with respect to any symptoms that may require diagnosis or medical attention.

For permission requests, write to the publisher, addressed "Attention: Permissions Coordinator," at the address below:

School Farm

Bentley Common

Warwickshire

England

CV9 2HP

Jeni@jenibennett.com

BONUS: Register as a Preferred Client with Arbonne and get up to 60% Discount on products mentioned in this book

To help you get the most out of this book and to turbo- charge your fitness and weight management efforts, I want to give you the best start you could have in supercharging your fitness & health.

Fit & Fab Forever in 90 Days: Tips, Tricks & Secrets Every Professional Woman Over 40 Can Start TODAY!

If you're looking to succeed with fitness & weight management then this brand new book by beauty, health, & wellness expert, Jeni Bennett, reveals how every Professional Woman Over 40 can understand how to get into the right mindset, what you've done wrong before and how you can do it right this time..

- An in-depth peek into Jeni's background with weight management (and how it holds the key to your success with the ability to manage you weight, tone your body and eat better in 90 days.)

- The "Million Dollar TIP" Jeni Bennett wishes someone had shared about weight management when she was first starting out (and the best way for Professional women over 40 put this tip into action today)
- A VERY cool TRICK Jeni figured out and discovered with weight management that will revolutionise the way Professional women over 40 succeed with the ability to manage you weight, tone your body and eat better in 90 days.
- The #1 SECRET every Professional Woman Over 40 needs to know when it comes to weight management (and why it's a secret most people have no clue about)
- Lots of other juicy tips, tricks & secrets about weight management all Professional women over 40 need to know about
- Specific tools for weight management all Professional women over 40 need to know about (so you can understand how to get into the right mindset, what you've done wrong before and how you can do it right this time.)
- How to develop the perfect mindset every Professional Woman Over 40 must have about weight management that virtually guarantees success
- And, as a special bonus, we'll also reveal the Plant based protein that will change your eating habits, that you can order and get delivered directly to your door!

So go ahead, click or the link right now and you're on your way to Fitness & weight management success!

http://www.jenibennett.arbonne.com

Table of Content

ATTENTION: A Special Note about how this book was created.

Dear Professional Woman Over 40,

Thank you for getting your copy of "Fit & Fab Forever in 90 Days - Weight Management Tips, Tricks & Secrets Every Professional Woman Over 40 can start TODAY!"

This book will teach you critical fitness & weight management skills, tools, techniques and more that every Professional Woman Over 40 needs to understand and apply.

This book was originally created as a live interview.

That's why it <u>reads as a conversation</u> rather than a traditional "book" that talks "at" you.

I wanted you to feel as though I am talking "with" you, much like a close friend or relative.

I felt that creating the material this way would make it easier for you to grasp the topics and put them to use quickly, rather than wading through hundreds of pages.

So relax.

Grab a pen or pencil and some paper to take notes.

And get ready to take your fitness & weight management to the next level so that you can understand how to get into the right mindset, understand what you've done wrong before and how you can do it right this time.

Let's get started with the ability to manage your weight, tone your body and eat better in 90 days.

Right now...

Sincerely yours,

Jeni Bennett

Meet Jeni Bennett

Jeni Bennett is an expert in fitness & weight management whose accomplishments include:

Education:

- B.Ed Hons Education
- Sales & Marketing Diploma
- AET Qualified
- Qualified Fitness Instructor
- Zumba Trained
- Zumba Burst - HIIT
- Zumba Glutes – FiTT
- Nutrition Diploma
- IDTA Dance Qualifications
- Makeup Artist Qualified
- Beauty Specialist Qualified
- Makeup Artist Trainer Qualified
- PhD From the School of Hard Knocks

Work History:

- Taught fitness & dance for over 25 years
- Created Charity Zumbathons and fundraiser events
- Worked as a LEA teacher and educator

- Experience Manager Level Consultant in Legal & Education Recruitment
- Spent nearly 20 years performing in theatres, TV shows, clubs and community events
- Member of the Guild of Beauty Therapists
- Owner of Savage Beauty Academy

Awards, Titles, and Designations:

- Award Winning Makeup Artist
- Mrs Warwickshire, 2017
- Crowned Mrs United Kingdom, 2017/18 aged 52years
- Crowned Mother of the Year, 2018 – Palm Springs
- Foster Mother of 21 children to date

Personal Info:

- Married to a Dairy Farmer, Michael
- Dancer on the 90's TV show 'Hitman & Her'
- Represented the United Kingdom in Palm Springs, USA 2018 at the Mrs Globe Pageant
- Worked two jobs whilst studying at university and a single parent to Domanique
- An Extra in **'The Feed'**
- Featured in **'This is Woman'** by Executive Producer **Russ Malkin** of Long Way Down with **Ewan McGregor** & more recently he directed films with **David Beckham** & **Prince Harry**

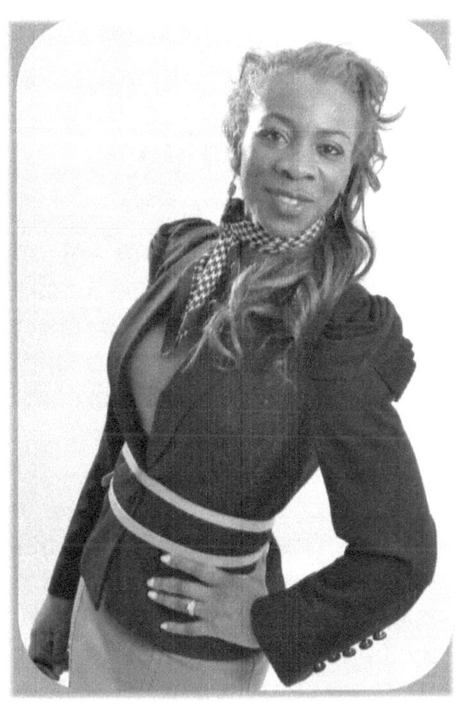

Ladies, most of what you need is instruction and encouragement from someone who has "been there and done that!" with how to get into the right mindset, what you've done wrong before and how you can do it right this time.

And as you can see, fitness & weight management expert Jeni Bennett is uniquely qualified to help you understand everything you need to know about the ability to manage your weight, tone your body and eat better in 90 days!

Introduction

Domanique: Okay then. Hi everyone and welcome to Fitness & Weight Management Tips, Tricks, and Secrets. Jeni Bennett reveals how every professional woman over 40 can get into the right mindset, what you've done wrong before, and how you can do it right this time.

My name is Domanique Savage-Ramsey and today I'm talking with fitness & weight management expert, Jeni Bennett about the tips, tricks, and secrets every professional woman over 40 needs to shortcut their way to success with weight management and get great results faster. So welcome Jeni Bennett.

Jeni Bennett: Thank you Domanique for having me. That's wonderful.

Domanique: Jeni is a well-known expert on the subject of weight management and has graciously consented to this interview to share with us all the cool tips and tricks that hardly any professional woman over 40 knows about that could really accelerate your results and help you with how to get into the right mindset, what you've done wrong before, and how you can do it right this time. So Jeni, thank you again for joining us for this live interview. Let's jump right in.

Jeni Bennett: Absolutely. I'm so thrilled to be here. OK, lets go.

Meet Your Fitness & Weight Management Expert, Jeni Bennett

Domanique: My first question is about your background and experience in the field of fitness & weight management so that the professional woman over 40 in our audience can understand who you are, where you're coming from, and how you can relate to where they are right now. And then we'll jump into the cool stuff with tips, tricks & secrets about the weight management so our audience can get the real inside scoop. So my first question, could you tell us a little bit about yourself in terms of background, education, and experience in fitness & weight management?

Jeni Bennett: Absolutely Domanique. Thank you. So I started off literally dancing out of my mummy's tummy I'm sure! I have always been very keen to be dancing. I took dancing up as a young child and I went on to become a student teacher with the IDTA. I then went on and did various dance shows and things like that. It was always on the dance side originally. Even when I went to university I actually thought I was going to do a PE & dance major; but I actually trained as a primary school teacher with history as my major. So actually there was a little bit of a change there

I just loved studying about history and finding out more.

I've since gone on to be qualified with an AET qualification. I'm a fully qualified fitness instructor with FITT & HIIT credentials. I have nutrition training & I'm a Zumba Gold Instructor.

In addition to this Domanique, I have full experience on the makeup and beauty side. They have always been of very keen interest to me so I am a fully-qualified makeup artist MGBT Member of the Guild of Beauty Therapists and A trained beauty specialist. I have a Beauty School and I now train makeup artists to qualify with full accreditation.

Finally Domanique, I can honestly say that I have a PhD from the school of hard knocks.

Domanique: Fantastic, Jeni. That's a phenomenal range of qualifications you have there. Tell us a bit about your experience please.

Jeni Bennett: Of course. So, besides working within local educational authorities as a teacher and an educator; my experience has been over 45 years within fitness and dance. I spent numerous years performing in theatres, TV shows, clubs & community events.

I am an avid philanthropist and I have created various charity events, such as Zumbathons, dance shows and even street dance performances. I actually set up a street dance academy for the youth in my local area. We performed in at community events and in front of the regional MP (Member of Parliament).

Domanique: Wow Jeni, you do keep yourself busy. So how have these qualifications and experiences been celebrated?

Jeni   Thank you Domanique! Well, I have won a number of awards for dance and fitness competitions. I'm an award-winning makeup artist and competed in a National Event at the NEC. In 2017 I was given the Title 'Mrs Warwickshire', for the charity & fundraising work I do. I then went on to be crowned' Mrs. United Kingdom 2017'. I was thrilled in June 2018 to be able to represent the UK in Palms Springs, USA at the grand age of 53 years, where I was given the accolade of 'Mother of the Year' because my husband & I have fostered 21 children over the last few years.

So Domanique, although all this may seem as though it has very little to do with fitness & weight management, it's to do with being a professional woman who runs several business, has an hectic life, but I still manage to find the time to write a book, support professional women in their quest to be fit and look fab. It's important that I share my tips, tricks & secrets of how a very busy professional woman can managing your weight, feel great, look fit and be fabulous even when you are over 40.

Domanique: That's brilliant. So you had a lot of formal education with regards to the weight management. Were you an overnight success or did you have to work for this?

Jeni Bennett: Oh my goodness, I was absolutely not an overnight success. It's taken years of dedication and getting the right qualifications; understanding the body; nutrition and all the rest of it to get on top of the fitness aspect.

So, it's important for me that people understanding as a busy professional woman, what it is like to run a family home, work several businesses, be present in my relationship with my husband and still help others find their time to **create the body they want to live in!**

I'm not an overnight successful Domanique; I have worked very hard at this.

Domanique: Okay, Jeni. Thank you.

Please tell my audience what kind of things do you feel or experience with regards to fitness & weight management that would be relevant to my audience of professional women over 40?

Jeni Bennett: Absolutely. Well the things that I've done that I feel are relevant are very much about understanding the body. The body changes as we get older, and as a professional woman, understanding that it's different when you're over 40 to when you're in your 20s.

Our bodies can't do the same thing in the same way. Post-partum, if we have had a baby, or several! If we gave birth naturally or via caesarean; Elderly primigravida; Osteoporosis, Arthritic pain, Sciatica can all affect women over 40 to varying degrees and are just a few of the issues that can occur which can make exercise more painful and uncomfortable.

Hormones, PMS, Female Incontinency, bladder weakness, hysterectomies and menopause all affect the female body differently.

Women can get trapped when the menopause kicks in. Those hot flushes can be hellish! The bed sheets and bedclothes can feel sopping wet from those night sweats; and you definitely don't want your other half to cuddle up to you.

I should know! Ha ha!

Even things like 'jumping jacks' can be so uncomfortable if you have bladder weakness. And I know that a lot of ladies find this a very uncomfortable exercise, but so many men still suggest we should do it! & that's because they have no idea what it is like to push a baby out, or have bladder weakness. It's a great full-body workout, but it's a terrible exercise if you're trying to hold your waters!

Domanique: Ha, Ha! Very good Jeni! Yeah!

Jeni Bennett: Well, Let's get down to the nitty gritty and say it as it is... When we were younger, losing weight was so much easier, we might decide to not have an extra bag of crisps, one less scoop of ice cream, run to catch the bus or decide to swim whilst at the gym. But, as our age goes up, Domanique, our metabolic rate decides to nose-dive; which means that what used to be a really good exercise & diet strategy, has suddenly become a major formula for serious weight gain.

As much as I hate to say it Domanique, for women specifically, hormonal changes after age 40, can make it so much harder to lose weight and keep it off. However, we don't have to buy a bigger wardrobe, just because we are getting older. Weight management after 40 is possible, and, even better, it doesn't have to be a struggle.

Domanique   Well Jeni, that's great but some ladies really do struggle with their weight after 40 and get stuck in a downward spiral or yo-yo diet, can you shed any light on how you can help them move forward please?

Jeni

Of course Domanique, that's what I'm here for. I'm going to give a very brief and generalised over view of **The Menopause**.

I had a hysterectomy aged 45 and I went into premature menopause straight away. I was offered HRT, but I felt this made me put on weight and I wanted to find out more about what was actually going on inside my body. I might have stopped having periods, but the hormonal changes and menopause were a nightmare!

First of all, I found out that as women become menopausal, they experience a number of symptoms, including menopausal weight gain. Now, while it is one of the more frustrating symptoms of menopause, it is also one of the most common. In fact, research has shown that up to 90% of menopausal women will experience weight gain at some level. And actually, putting on weight is a normal and common aspect of getting older. By us, better understanding why it is likely to happen, during menopause, women can put things in place to manage their menopausal weight gain.

Another fact that made me want to find out more about weight gain and the menopause Domanique, was that women who increase their weight by in excess of 20 pounds (20lbs) after menopause are likely to increase their breast cancer risk by nearly 20%, but those who lose 20 pounds after menopause are able to reduce their breast cancer risk by as much as 23%

Domanique   So why are women more likely to put on this extra weight Jeni?

Jeni   Here are some facts about the menopause and our hormonal changes:

Estrogen or Oestrogen - Primary female sex hormone, it is responsible for the development and regulation of the female reproductive system. As a woman's ovaries produce less estrogen, her body attempts to draw from other sources of estrogen. Fat cells can produce estrogen, so her body works harder to convert calories into fat to increase estrogen levels. Unfortunately, fat cells do not burn calories the way muscle cells do, which causes weight gain.

Progesterone - Water retention is often linked to menopause because water weight and bloating can result from a decrease in progesterone levels. Though this doesn't actually result in weight gain, clothes can feel a bit tighter and a woman may feel uncomfortable in her clothes and think she's heavier.

Testosterone – This male hormone increases at the onset of menopause. It's responsible for redistributing weight to the midsection instead of to the hips.

Did you know? Most women experience a 5% decrease in metabolic rate each decade. So, because metabolism slows as we women approach menopause, we need about **200 less calories** a day to maintain our weight as we enter our mid to late 40s.

I personally use a supplement called **Arbonne Essentials Daily Power Packs For Women, with Vitamins & Minerals.** It is an excellent source of 20 vitamins & minerals that include: Vitamin A, B6, B12, C, D, E, Thiamine, Riboflavin, Folate, Calcium, Magnesium and you can get it too via my link www.jenibennett.arbonne.com

Well, as a woman's estrogen & progesterone decreases, sometimes by 40 – 60%, so our appetite can cause us to eat more. There has even been a study that shows women can eat up to 67% more than they would before the menopause. So this upsurge in appetite together with a sluggish metabolism with the onset of menopause can cause weight gain in women. This could, perhaps, account for the 12% jump in the number of women who become overweight during midlife compared to women in their 20's and 30's.

A Fitness & Weight Management Tip I Wish I'd Know Way Back When...

Domanique: Yeah, okay. Well it's obvious that you're an expert for fitness & weight management so let's get down to the tips, tricks and secrets. What is a tip you wish someone had shared with you about fitness & weight management when you were first starting out and why would this tip be so valuable?

Jeni Bennett: Absolutely. We all know about drinking less alcohol, doing more exercise, eating better. But one of the main things is to stand up. It might not be dancing but literally, think about this; professional women may be ... sleeping for eight hours a day if we're lucky! Most women sleep a lot less.

But in 24 hours if you sleep eight hours a day, then you might be sitting at your desk, in meetings, etc. for maybe 7 to 10 hours some days.

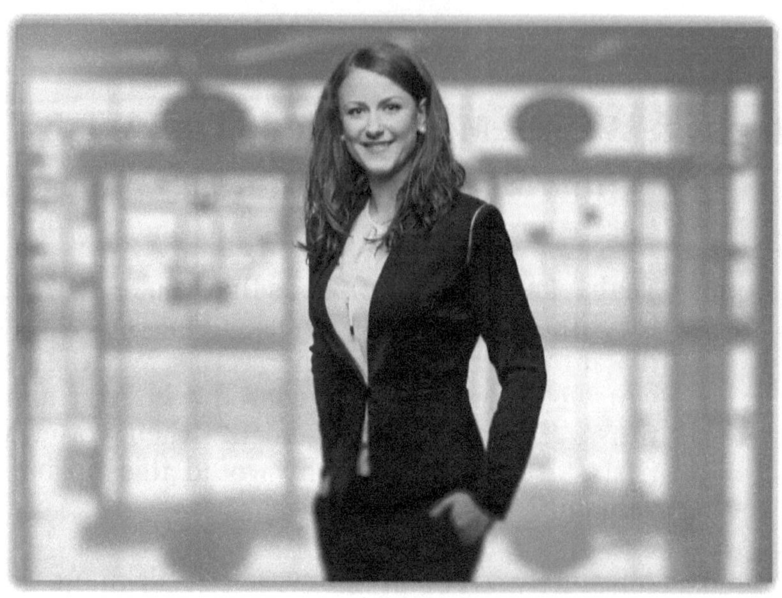

Then as a Professional Woman, you could be commuting or driving, to work, this might take up another couple of hours a day...

You might go home and relax in front of the TV or go out for a meal or whatever you do in the evening and again you're sitting down.

That's a lot of time sitting!

Stand up.

Stand up on your feet.

Sitting on the train, plane or automobile; sitting in meetings, sitting at your desk, sitting for lunch, dinner, restaurant, sitting for a after work drink, sitting watching the TV, at the movies... WOW! This means that most of us get into the very sedentary lifestyle because we are not active enough.

Our bodies were made as human beings to be active. Whether it's searching for food or fuel; our body was made to be physically active making our dwellings habitable, building, cooking, creating and killing to survive... Well, we might not live in the Stone Ages anymore and need to go out and hunt for our food, but back in those days, most people were considered old if you reached 40 years on this earth!

Anyway, Domanique well regarded nutritionist **Lisa Jubilee** says that one way to burn more calories daily is to stand more and sit less. And I absolutely agree.

British studies have shown that we burn about 50 calories an hour just by standing. So we actually can lose weight standing up more... think about that. Lose 50 calories just standing up for an hour. So three hours a day that's 150. Now every year if we did that each day at work, that's 30,000 extra calories just by standing. That's eight pounds (8lbs) you could lose of fat by just standing up more often. Now if you stand up and dance, wow, just imagine.

So I suggest Domanique, that my first tips is to ask all those professional women over 40 to stand up at work, stand up in the home, stand up on the train... Just stand ladies.

Whether it's standing on the bus or whether it's standing at the office. But if you can stand for about three hours a day and you can do some movements while you're standing, burn those calories. So that I think is a great tip, I wish I knew about when I was working in an office Domanique.

Domanique: Yeah, it sounds as though there's lots of different ways that professional women can put this tip into action Jeni. Do you feel there might be any other tips on this... it sounds pretty straightforward?

Jeni Bennett: I think basically you've got to just stand on your own two feet.

Domanique: Yeah, your right Jeni, we need to stand on our feet, possibly in sensible shoes, right!

Jeni Bennett: Yeah, ha-ha, you can do it immediately. It's something that you can implement straightaway. Bare feet, high heels or trainers! Right?

Domanique: Yeah.

Jeni Bennett: It's not an idea that you need to think about. So sometimes people get stuck around what can I do that's immediate and quick? Well that's something you can do straight off the bat. You can do it today. In a year you can be half a stone lighter!

Domanique   Is there another tip you can give us at this point please Jeni?

Jeni   **Pelvic Floor Muscles**

We've got to start squeezing!

We spoke about 'Jumping Jacks' earlier and how they can be really uncomfortable for women over 40. We were all told about this as teens, or when we went to maternity classes; but I am shocked as to how many women have incontinence issues when they sneeze, laugh, cough, get stressed, lift something heavy or just can't hold it. The main causes of bladder weakness, pelvic prolapse or incontinence are **Neurological damage, Medical conditions, Menopause and Pregnancy.**

As a women over 40, we can have a prolapse of this pelvic muscle area which can lead to all sorts of medical issues later on in life, and it is a little known fact that incontinence pads have become some of the highest selling feminine hygiene products in the 2010's, with 1:4 women suffering from either stress, urge or mixed incontinence

Domanique, let me tell you that it is important to know what sort of issue you might be dealing with, because if you know that you're dealing with **stress incontinence**, you can gain a lot by doing 'clenches' or 'squeeze exercises' on a regular basis. But if you have **urge incontinence**, you need to practice filling your bladder and developing that muscle (because the bladder is a muscle)!

So that you can increase the bladder's ability to hold water and over time you will lengthen the amount of time between emptying intervals.

Domanique   Ok Jeni, so you're saying that you can help women who are suffering from bladder weakness or pelvic floor issues to regain their ability to strengthen this muscle. Now, that's a fitness guru achievement if ever there was one.

Jeni   Well yes Domanique, there are several ways for a woman to strengthen her pelvic floor muscles to support the bladder.

For **Stress Incontinence**, when you are in the car whilst driving, on the train when commuting, at the desk whilst working, even in a meeting, at the bar or whilst making love! We can strengthen our pelvic floor and develop that muscle by doing the 'squeeze, squeeze, squeeze, release, rest, start again!' exercise.

For **Urge Incontinence**, you need to drink plenty of water throughout the day, hold your water 15 minutes longer each time before you go to the toilet. When you are there you need to do what I teach some of my foster children, which are that after you have gone 'count to 10 and try again!'

In addition to these, reducing caffeine and tobacco intake is also highly recommended as these substances can worsen incontinence. Health professionals also recommend continuing your pelvic floor exercises (Kegels) and ensuring you maintain a healthy weight.

Domanique   Fantastic Jeni, that was a brilliant tip, can you give us another?

Jeni   **Pepper, Black Pepper to be precise!**

Did you know Domanique, that seasoning can be the main event when it comes to weight management? I'm sure all you ladies have heard about the amazing fat-burning properties of cayenne or turmeric, right? but I have to say there is a silent hero when it comes to spices that burn fat. And that is the one and only partner to salt; that's right the humble black pepper.

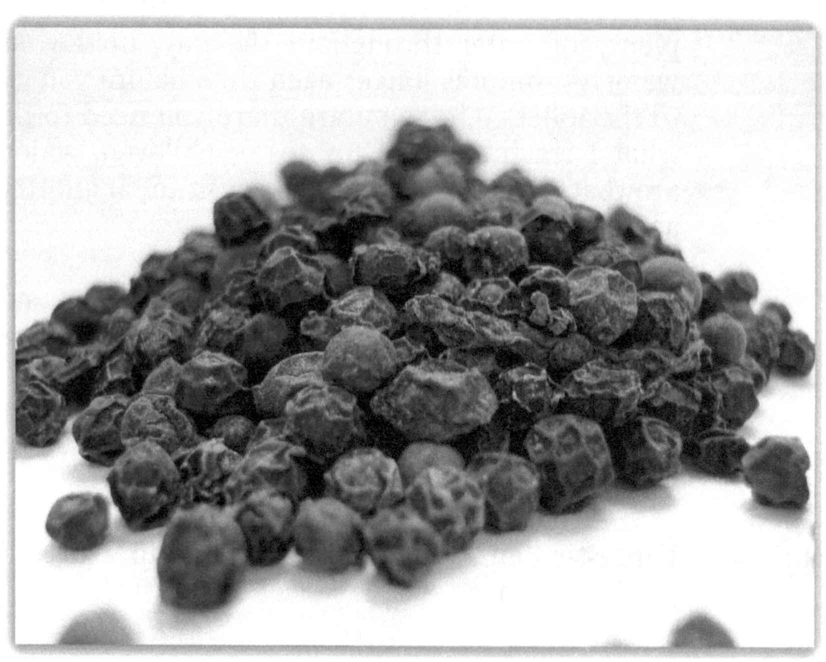

Used in Eastern medicine for centuries, **Black pepper** contains a compound called **piperine**, it is used to treat ailments such as upset stomachs as well as inflammation. In fact, Scientists have found that piperine's anti-inflammatory properties could even extend to preventing new fat cells from forming. Yes ladies, the meek stuff sitting unnoticed on a table near you could be the answer to bowel, inflammation & fat cells issues!

So, cook with herbs and spices, don't over spice your food with chillies that will disrupt the bowel.

Cut down your salt intake by substituting flavourful herbs for salt. Adding black pepper, spices and herbs to foods can also help you enjoy eating healthy food!

How's that for a tip... use more black pepper.

A Cool Fitness & Weight Management Trick I Figured Out

Domanique: Yes. Okay, that's amazing Jeni, who knew?

So, my next question, what is a cool trick you figured out or discovered with fitness & weight management that would really help the professional woman over 40 in our audience with the ability to manage their weight, tone their body and eat better in 90 days?

Jeni Bennett: **Shop Online**

Absolutely! Well I would say one of the best tricks that professional women could do is get our food delivered. We are busy women! We have a lot of things going on. One of the reasons why I say this is, shopping online means you can organise your week, decide what you want to cook, make or bake each week and then do it!

If you have your food delivered, you can go online; get your weeks' worth of ingredients. You can then create your own salads, sandwiches, soups, pack lunches, pasta meals. You can get them all sorted for yourself, your husband & children. By purchasing your food online, you are much less tempted to buy unhealthy foods. Those additional cakes, crisps, sweets and treats at the checkout counter will no longer haunt you... bit of this, lots of that; it stops you putting in extra ingredients in your basket that you actually either don't use or don't need.

In addition to this, and I love this aspect, when you're online, you can see the calories, fat content, sugar level, cholesterol, fibre, protein and so much more.

By shopping online, you can create the healthiest version of yourself, because you can get your carbs and get your proteins in. Get your milks and dairies in. If you're intolerant you can get the right gluten-free, lactose-free, sugar-free based foods. But how amazing is it to be able to do all of that online.

Set it up for the week.

Get it delivered directly to you.

You then don't have to think about going to the store, because one of the key things I find people do, especially busy, professional women; is they don't have time to make breakfast, so they go without.

They don't have time for lunch because they have to go to a meeting, so they go to the service station or the petrol station to grab a sandwich

(450), a packet of crisps (189), a muffin (427) and a drink (150) which could potentially contains 100% of their daily calorific intake. They then eat whilst sitting at their desk or on their way to a meeting and that don't feel full, because most of these are 'empty calories'!

You're going to be thinking, 'I don't feel full'. You're going to think, 'I've only had a snack'. You haven't got the right energy. You probably have a sugar spike because you're not eating healthy. You're grabbing on the hoof and it's one of the worst things to do.

Or just as bad is asking a colleague to pick you up something whilst their out at lunch. It is the worst way of eating and unfortunately as a busy professional woman over 40, you're going to find that by eating on the go, you're adding calories daily rather than losing them. You're hindering your healthy eating by doing that.

When you buy your weekly meals online, you can now make time to create your own beautiful meals that they've cooked or made. You will know exactly what's in it! You can pre-make and bulk freeze pasta, home-made sauces; frozen fruit & vegetables; even cheese, cooked meats, fish dishes, chillies dishes or protein shakes and much more.

And so that for me is one of the key tricks Domanique.

Reformulate your shopping habits to help you readjust your mindset and help you create the eating habits that will help you become fit and manage your weight.

Domanique: Okay. And if someone gets stuck on this trick, how can they get unstuck?

Jeni Bennett: Well, I think the key thing is you set up your account and get started.

So sometimes people get stuck in the thought process of…"Well, I haven't got time to do it!" My answer is to help my clients find the 'white spaces' in their calendar to do this. I help them look at when they currently do their shopping. Do they have time to go to the supermarket, local store or at lunch time, if you've got time to put those things in the basket and if you're doing that every lunch time, or every week, then you are wasting valuable time, so you defiantly have time to set up your online shopping account.

Once it's done, most online shopping carts let you reorder every week, fortnight or monthly. You can add to it and take things away; but at least you can see exactly what you're buying. One of the things that I do with my clients is make sure that they empty their fridge, their pantry, their freezer of all the rubbish that they are not going to eat over the next 90 days, that's either not good for them or that's been at the back of the shelf etc.

You can make your own soup. You can make your own salad. You can get yourself started and I think as a trick, get that trick in place and it gets you unstuck and it gets you set up immediately to eat right and to eat well. When you do this, my clients are surprised with how much time they have available to eat well, tone the body and feel fab. They manage their weight much better **Refocus** their old habit into a new healthy one that supports them and their family.

I do get asked by some people if they can still shop at & support their local store; and I have to say YES! I have a fantastic local store who will put my shopping list together for me to collect on my way home from work every week. In fact they love this, because they know that I am a loyal customer and I will do everything I can to support them.

Finally on this Domanique, I want to say that there are a number of 'ready packaged healthy meal' companies out there that also deliver a weeks' worth of ingredients or ready-made meals to you and for some of my ladies, this absolutely is the way to go! Not only do you know exactly what's in the meal, but you get everything fresh and as a busy professional woman, this has got to be an advantage

Domanique: Thank you for this Jeni, are there any other amazing tricks at this point with fitness & weight management we need to let professional women over 40 know about?

Jeni Bennett: **Buy new plates – size matters!**

That's right, I know that there is a 'thing' at the moment about having these extra-large plates, but come on ladies; do we need to fill them with food? Big portions have become the norm, both when eating out and at home.

Go out today and buy new plates! Healthy eating can start with buying new crockery. Using smaller plates to cut back on your portion sizes can be helpful. Ditch the 12-inchers and start using the 9-inch ones. A swap like this can add up to major calorie cutbacks.

In a study carried out at **Cornell University**, reducing your plate size from 30cm to 25cm led to 22% less calories being consumed. This may seem strange, but eating your meals on a smaller plate can also be much more fulfilling than a large plate that's half empty!

Portion Distortion is a real thing and I truly believe that **you shape** your body with the activities you do, but **you size** your body in the kitchen & the amount of food you eat.

A Secret Every Professional Woman Over 40 Needs To Know

Domanique: Okay, so what is a secret every professional woman over 40 needs to know when it comes to fitness & weight management?

Jeni Bennett: Never, Ever, Ever make weight management or fitness a 'New Year Resolution'!

It is one of the biggest mistakes adults make and one of the greatest secrets the Fitness Industry know works in their favour every year.

Men & women decide to eat & drink in excess over the whole of December, when you start getting invitations to the various works Christmas parties. You then arrange to meet up with old friends, for a drink or two. You go to visit family, or they come to you and you all have the most enormous Christmas Eve, Christmas Day, Boxing Day, New Year's Eve, New Year Day meals, which tend to be high in fat, sugar, cholesterol, carbohydrates & alcohol whilst even the vegetables are smothered in butter, sauces or hidden amongst breadcrumbs or under gravy!

You then book to go to the gym and pay a year's subscription (money in the gyms bank account gaining interest) or monthly for a set period!

You have all the best intentions when you start going to the gym at the beginning of January. They are packed, everyone is motivated, and gyms are at their largest capacity on the 2nd week of January. You feel you can start making a difference to your body, this is great, this is what you want...

Then somehow you miss a session here and a session there and by the 14th of February, Valentine's Day, You stop attending altogether! **Research has shown that some 80% of the New Year's Resolutions gym-bunnies stop going by the second week of February.** So, Just 20% of people who started going to the gym only 6 weeks ago Domanique, are still using their membership; that's ridiculous isn't it?

Domanique   I really didn't know it was so few Jeni, that's crazy. So how can Professional Women, over 40 get around this secret the companies have been keeping from us?

Jeni   Well, I suggest to my clients to start their fitness and weight management with me any month, but not January! This might sound strange, but the secret is to be Fit & Fab Forever! not just for 6 weeks and stop.

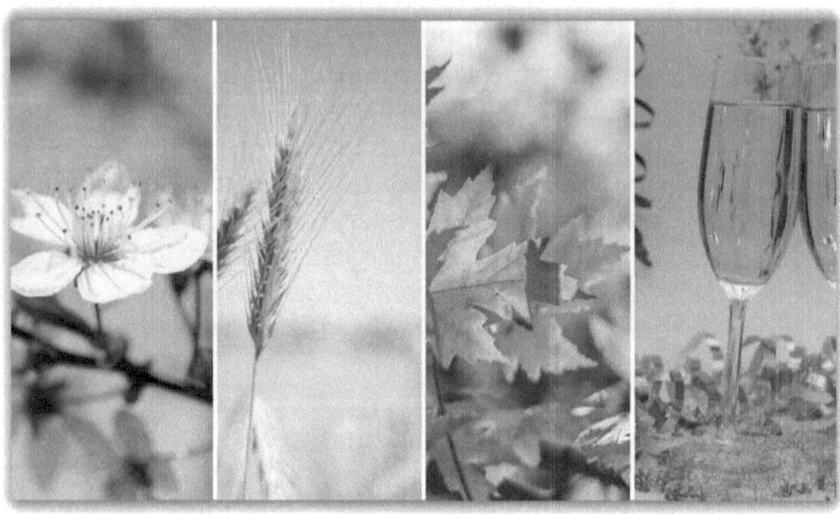

Start in September, October or November to look stunning & create an healthy eating habit ready for over the Christmas period.

Start in February, March or April to be gorgeous with a summer beach body everyone will envy.

Start in June, July or August if you want to stay away from the crowds, because the gyms are near empty at this time of year.

By doing this you would have trained yourself into a better understanding of eating and fitness habits. You will have learnt a lot about yourself and what you can do daily to achieve the goal you want.

You will be well on your way to *'create the body you want to live in'*... and therefore, you are less likely to pile on the pounds over the festive season or whilst on that all-inclusive Summer, Autumn, Winter or Spring break.

Start in January if you must, but not as a New Year's resolution, don't fall for the hype. Gyms know that they typically sell new memberships with the probability that a just 20% of people will actually use them. This means there is only a 1:5 chance you'll use yours consistently for longer than two months.

Finally on this Domanique, I have an amazing program called **'30 Days To Healthy Living & Beyond'** that helps kick start my female clients. We have a monthly reset boot-camp and it's amazing way to reset your body!

Domanique: Okay Jeni. Are there any other secrets that you can tell us about weight management and the ability to be fitter and more fabulous forever?

Jeni Bennett: Yes, Domanique. A major secret out there is that 'healthy foods are not always healthy'!

I was shocked when I was undertaking my nutritional training to note that most products that are labelled healthy, natural or skinny; were not actually the best food for me or my clients. In fact some of them you might as well be eating a slab of fudge, placed between two cookies, topped with loads of whipped cream and dripping with chocolate... Especially if you buy American packaged products, because you do not have to prove that a product is 'natural' 'healthy' or 'nutritional' before you label it and the stores stock it! Crazy hey!

Now I have nothing against USA, but their labelling laws are not as strictly regulated as the UK & Europe, so food manufacturers can literally put whatever *buzz words* they think will connect with their customers and drive up their sales.

Remember this; the healthiest foods don't usually need labelling, because they are fresh, eg berries, eggs, meat, fruits or vegetables!

For example, did you know – peanut butter, grapes, bananas, eggs, rice, herbal teas, yogurt and hard cheese can all help reduce gas and fight bloating?

However, there are several foods most people think are healthy and they are not as healthy as you might think.

Here are my Top 8 healthy, NOT healthy **foods:**

Energy Bars	Energy = Sugar! When it comes to these bars, most are loaded with hidden sugar, fat, calories & artificial ingredients. Please read the label closely if you really want an 'energy bar'! Opt for low in sugar, high in fibre & protein. Make sure you can understand and recognise the ingredients... OR Make your own.
Whole Wheat Bread	Renowned, Miami clinical nutritionist **Dr. Michael Forman** said that 'Whole wheat bread is considered one of the most potentially inflammatory foods in existence since the gluten used in today's wheat bread is virtually indigestible by most people,' It can also raise blood sugar which makes you more likely to store fat.
Fruit Juice	Fruit juices have high sugar content and zero fibre, resulting in a spike in blood sugar. **Nutritionist Jennifer Keirstead,** suggests that Instead of fruit juice, opt for fruit smoothies, which do have fibre. When possible, cut sugar levels by working in some vegetables.
Soy Milk	If you get congested, suffer from inflammation or don't wish to eat GMO or estrogenic foods, then you may wish to stay away from Soy milk. It is described as being worse that cow's milk. Research has shown that Soy milk is a highly processed. For non-dairy sources of calcium

	try some leafy greens such as kale & bok-choy, almonds, oranges, seaweed and canned salmon.
Skimmed Milk	"Skim dairy isn't healthy and it's not good for your weight," says **Lauren Slayton, MS, RD, and founder of Foodtrainers**. When you cut out all the fats in milk you're left with a large amount of androgens (hormones). Instead opt for low-sugar, full-fat, coconut milk, almond milk or rice milk.
Tofu	Did you know that Tofu acts as an estrogen-like substance causing all kinds of bodily havoc; apparently, it's one of the **10 foods that can cause man-boobs!** 90% or more of Soy products are GMO which means that they can withstand intense chemical sprays meant to destroy plants, So think about this, if the powerful chemicals can't destroy the plant, how does your body break down & digest it?
Granola	Full of sugar... way too much sugar. Instead of granola try some Greek yogurt, topped with seeds, nuts, chai and berries. Or cooked unsweetened oatmeal or sugar-free flakes. If you want more sweetness try dried or frozen fruit but make sure you're picking dried fruit with no added sugar, sulphites, preservatives or other additives.
Flavoured Yogurt	Most flavoured yogurts have far too much sugar to be beneficial. The flavouring is actually sweet, sugar loaded gelatine that makes flavoured yogurt very fattening. High in calories, with low if any fibre.

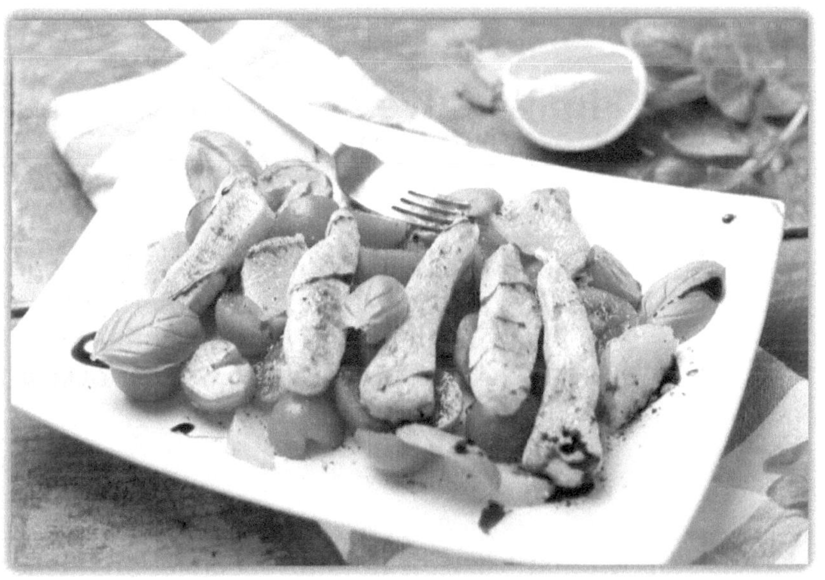

More Juicy Fitness & Weight Management Tips, Tricks & Secrets

Domanique: Oh my goodness Jeni, I didn't know that about flavoured yogurt. So are there any other juicy tips or secrets at this point with weight management we need to let our professional women over 40 know about?

Jeni Bennett: Yes, Domanique. **Eat frozen fruits**. Now this is a great tip, trick & secret. First of all, studies have shown that frozen fruit and vegetables are higher in nutrition because they are picked at the peak of the season and frozen immediately. So while fresh fruit are picked, packed, stored, shipped, stored, transported and then in the shop, this can actually take several weeks before we even get it.

Although I'm by no means advocating any one cutting out fresh fruit or vegetable; not at all!

What I do suggest is that you consider using frozen fruit & vegetables which are picked and frozen at their peak. Therefore, the nutritional content is higher; and the fruit or veg is definitely fresher.

If you love smoothies the way I love smoothies, or if you do protein shakes, or if you're creating your overnight oats or making a dessert, then get some frozen fruit. I tell you what; Putting frozen fruits into your smoothie is brilliant because you're not adding bare ice which only waters down the flavour. The smoothie is much thicker. You've got more nutrients in there and it really adds bulk to the actual creamy body of the final product.

Domanique: Okay, Jeni, that's fab. Is there any more you would like to add to this juicy piece of information?

Jeni Bennett: Yes, Domanique, as a Farmer's wife, I really have to say that I fully support the local farm producers, local farm shops and those restaurants & eateries who recognise food miles. Because this all means that we are reducing carbon omissions and purchasing at source where ever possible, which helps our local Farmers and producers.

Jeni Bennett

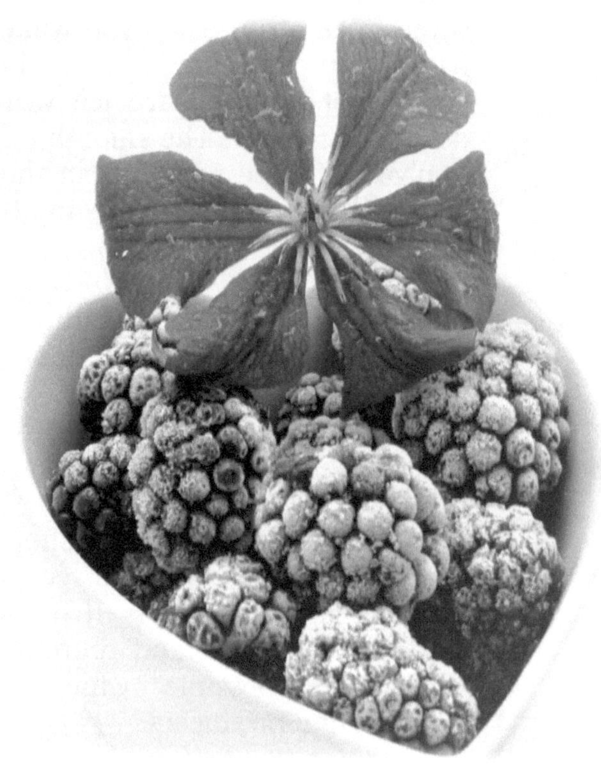

How It's Easier To Get Started With The Ability To Manage Your Weight, Tone Your Body And Eat Better In 90 Days. Today!

Domanique: Yeah. Is there anything I haven't asked you about fitness & weight management and the ability to manage your weight, trim your body and eat better in 90 days that you'd like to share with our audience of professional women over 40?

Jeni Bennett: Yes. What I'm going to add to this is actually about underwear / undergarments. It might sound like an interesting one but not many professional women are going to leave the house without a bra on! That is a given. But, they leave the house without good undergarments. And I tell you what, one of the best ways of feeling fab, looking toned and appearing as though you've lost some weight instantly is by having great undergarments.

If you've got a nice business dress or business suit and your bulky areas aren't being kept under control, get some great undergarments. It pulls, lifts, gives great curves and makes you look thinner and this can give you great confidence when you're in a meeting, going for an interview or presenting as a trainer or key note speaker.

There are some brilliant items out there these days that literally add to a woman's physique and I think, just as you wouldn't go out without a bra and feel confident, I don't think you should go out without good undergarments as a woman over 40, a professional woman or otherwise.

As a UK size 8 female, I love the lift, curves and toned effect I get when I wear quality undergarments. Leave the G-strings to the under 30's, give me great support any day! I think it helps me look stunning and I think it just adds to the whole ensemble!

Come on ladies, it's so easy to start '**creating the body you want to live in!'**

More Juicy Fitness & Weight Management Tips, Tricks & Secrets

Domanique | Jeni, Are there any other juicy tips, tricks & secrets at this point with Fitness & Weight management we need to let our Professional women over 40 know about?

Jeni | **Keep your hands busy**

When I was growing up, I was always told these two sayings

'The devil makes work for idle hands'

'Idle hands are the devils playthings'

I believe this to be true when it comes to weight management. Keeping your hands physically busy with activities such as adult colouring, knitting, crosswords, origami and even those fidget spinners, can prevent you from reaching for the closest fatty, salty or sugary snacks.

Stop spending hours watching the TV & munching away... Instead, take up a hobby that will give your hands and brain something to work together on. It might be flower arranging, gaming, writing your book, learning sign language, sewing or crafting. You decide, but get busy.

In fact, several studies of research have suggested that using your hands to **fidget** throughout the day can burn upwards of 300 calories, making it easier to slim down.'

The official term for fidgeting is actually **NEAT - Non-Exercise Activity Thermogenesis**, and is described as any moving about that isn't intended as a workout. So even things like using a fidget cube, taping a pencil, snapping a pen, swaying back and forth when you're standing, using your hands when you're speaking, tapping feet, clicking you fingers, and even twirling your hair are all examples of NEAT.

One study showed that slim people can fidget for about 150 minutes a day more than obese people do. These small, jittery actions have been shown to burn about 300 calories a day, which is equivalent to 10-30 (lbs) pounds a year!

Fitness & Weight Management Tools You Do NOT Need Anymore (Save Your Money)

Domanique Jeni, What are some Fitness & weight management tools, products or resources you think have become or are becoming obsolete? What or who is on the way out?

Jeni Well Domanique, I believe that 'artificial sweeteners' have had their day and are actually doing a disservice to the weight management industry. **Yale University** have produced research that has shown a link between artificial sweeteners, increase belly fat and risk of obesity.

In addition, sweeteners have been found to trigger hot flashes in women, so skip the sweeteners, loss the pounds and keep cool.

Domanique Thank you Jeni, any more?

Jeni Yes, now I don't believe that cocktails are ever going to go out of fashion, but I hope that women who are trying to manage their weight start to consider saying 'goodbye' to sugary happy hour drinks!

Did you know Domanique that a single flavoured cocktail or blended drink can have up to 600 calories per 8oz (8 ounce). So there are 2 reasons for not having these, firstly if you have two drinks, you've nearly had your day's intake of calories! Secondly, for menopausal women, this can dilate the blood vessels and cause further hot flashes.

Instead, go for my favourite tipple; **Champagne Ultra Brut** OR **Prosecco Brut**. Because ultra-brut is the driest of drinks & it is like saying 'no added sugar'. And that means fewer calories in your drink. What doesn't count, however, is serving your Champagne as a Mimosa, which will cut your alcohol content in half, but fill it up with even more sugary liquids.

Other alcoholic drinks that can be consumed whilst you're looking to manage your weight are: (a) **Tequila on the rocks** (with ice). You can sip, enjoy its smooth taste and nurse your drink over the evening. (b) **Vodka with a splash of soda**, which is better than tonic for calories. (c) Glass of **Wine**, which contains no wheat, so it won't make you feel bloated; moreover, red wine contains tannins, which in moderation, is good for your heart; polyphenols (a type of antioxidant) & is also prevalent in champagne. So like champagne, reds are linked to lowering blood pressure, improving cardiovascular health, and lessening the effects of free radical damage.

Avoid These Time Wasting Traps With The Ability To Manage Your Weight, Tone Your Body And Eat Better In 90 Days.

Domanique
: Where do you see Professional women over 40 wasting a lot of time in Fitness & weight management?

Jeni
: I wish more women would hold their personal self-care sacred to them and look after themselves more. I see too many women running about like 'Blue-ass Flies' and put so little time into getting enough sleep & active rest.

Getting a good night's sleep is one of life's greatest pleasures, and also a surprisingly effective means of slimming down. The results of the **Nurses' Health Study** reveal that, among a group of 60,000 women studied for 16 years, those who got 5 hours of sleep or less at night increased their risk of becoming obese by 15%. Getting adequate rest can also reduce your risk of dementia, according to **researchers at Johns Hopkins Bloomberg School of Public Health.**

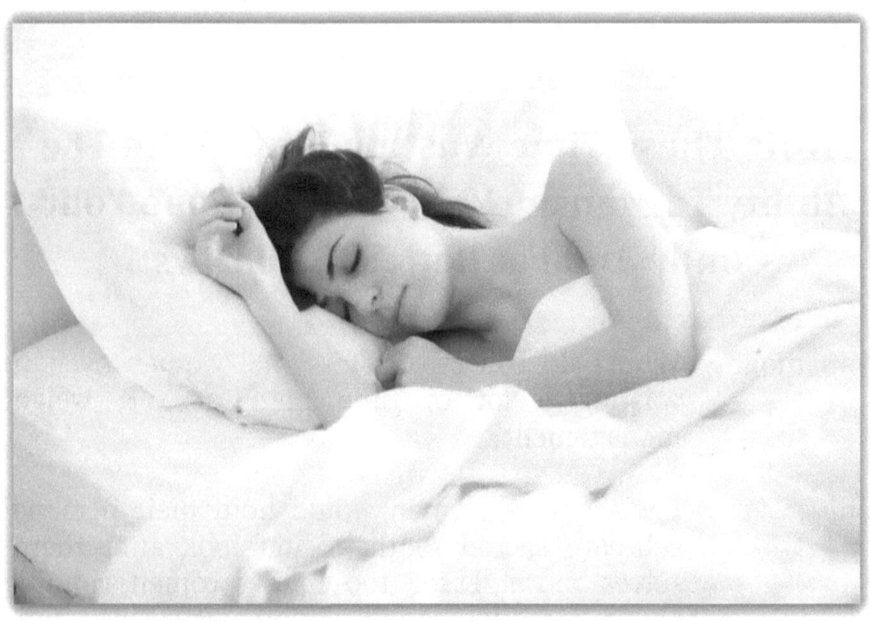

As a professional woman, you may be eating late due to meetings, entertaining clients or you may have children! If you do eat late at night, keep your portions small. And make sure that your last meal is at least a couple of hours before going to bed.

Active rest may include yoga, meditation, reflection, journaling, light music, reading etc. So spend time relaxing.

My Top 8 Tips to get a good night sleep are:

- Use blackout curtains
- Don't eat chocolate just before bedtime
- Have a warm shower or bath
- Drink a cup of mint or green tea rather than hot chocolate
- Don't sleep with the phone in your bedroom
- Put away your laptop or ipad a good hour before bedtime
- Don't sleep with the TV on; in fact no TV in the bedroom!
- Make love before bedtime!

A Cool Story About The Ability To Manage Your Weight, Tone Your Body And Eat Better In 90 Days.

Domanique   Jeni, I would really appreciate it if you could let my audience know if there one particular story, case study, or example you'd like to share that really sums up what we've been talking about here?

Jeni   Sure Domanique, I am very happy to give you an example of an amazing lady who I was working with for something else. She sits on a number of high level boards around female entrepreneurship, including one that advises government, she is a successful business owner and she travels the globe for meetings, work and conferences on a regular basis. Her life is busy and challenging so getting a balanced health and wellness regime was not an easy project!

At the initial consultation, she said she felt 'flabby' and wanted to lose about two stones. She was keen to get into a particular dress she wore for her engagement photoshoot and would love to be able to get into it again before her anniversary. In fact she sent me a picture of her trying to get it on and it would not zip up past her belly.

Domanique   OK, Jeni, this sounds intriguing!

Jeni   Yes, it was. Our first task was to **REFOCUS** her mindset and help her adjust to her reasons WHY she wanted to manage her weight. This was not a quick fix and so she had to carve out & protect the 'white space' in her calendar. Initially, she was asked to look at 4 x 2.5 minutes a day x 6 days a week.

She then needed to **REDEFINE** what her ideal weight, eating habits and lifestyle needs would be in the time period we were seeking to work in. We had to look at what *she said* she was physically doing and eating 'v' the reality of what she was actually doing and eating. The choices she was making in her basket whilst shopping; the snacks and treats she was purchasing, the times of day she was eating and the actual physical activities she was undertaking.

Although my client was jet-setting around the globe, working long hours and had a dog, which she walked daily; we had to **REACTIVATE** her momentum from a sedentary fitness routine that was not pushing her energy levels, heart rate, strength or stamina, consequently she was not using as much energy as she was consuming and therefore, the weight was not reducing and there was a lack of muscle tone in all areas. We looked at her ability to undertake 10 minutes of exercise a day... that's right, just 10 minutes a day of HIIT to deliver zone specific targeted muscle tone and strength. She must add other activities to this.

When I work with a client, I not only make sure that we undertake weight, height, BMI, standing pulse, and active pulse rates; we also take full body measurements, dietary requirements, known allergies, female conditions including; giving birth, it this was natural or assisted via caesarean; if she has had a hysterectomy and any other medical or physical issues that could affect her ability to complete the course.

I have a 'take no prisoners' attitude, when it comes to helping my clients and this really helped her become 'unstuck' when she was struggling with several issues and started to concentrate more on major calorie reduction, than healthy eating, (which was not appropriate for her body needs).

Domanique   So Jeni, can you go into a little more detail on this? When you say she needed to get 'unstuck' what do you mean?

Jeni   Unfortunately, sometimes, some of my clients start reverting back to their old ways of weight management or things they did in their younger days and end up either putting on weight or remaining static for a period!

They decide to cut calories, cut out meals and even fast; they over do certain exercises and cause themselves more harm than good.

I really hate when this happens.

I assist them in **REFORMULATING** their eating habits, to deliver a very target specific weight management and fitness program that gives them clear guidance that will leave them in no doubt as to what direction they need to be going in.

We revisit her goals as agreed at the beginning of the program. We reminded ourselves of what weight management she has undertaken before, what she felt worked and what didn't. We look at why she believes that this program will help her.

Finally she must decide to **REFOCUS** again on the Fit & Fab Forever approach of managing her weight, and I have to say Domanique; I have not failed with a single client who has continued with my strategies.

Domanique   So, how did this client fair Jeni?

Jeni   Well, the final part of my program is to **REALISE!** Realise that she has got this weight management & fitness thing 'in the bag!'

             She must realise that the only person who can put the food into her mouth is herself.

Realise that should she choose to drink alcohol, she needs to make good positive & knowledgeable decisions about what she has. Fitness and exercise comes in all shapes and sizes and the 10 minute a day mean that she can realise that it doesn't take much to tone her muscles, and reduce the fat.

So, of course she not only lost the 28lbs she was desperate to get rid of, but she also lost a few pound more!

She had a much better food management regime, because she took guidance on her fridge, freezer and store cupboard goods.

Finally she recovered the 'white space' in her calendar for herself and was able to work with her hectic schedule to ensure that she could pre-make meals to freeze and take to work, or have ready when she came home from work. She now had time to eat appropriate healthy and nutritious meals that were prepared in a timely manner. She was also able to secure her exercise time in order to achieve her goal

Domanique   And I'm sure we all want to know, did she get into her 10 year old body hugging dress?

Jeni   Oh YES!

She even took a picture and sent it to me with it fully zipped up

Time Management Tricks For How To Get Into The Right Mindset, What You've Done Wrong Before And How You Can Do It Right This Time.

Domanique   Any tips for time management when it comes to Fitness & weight management, please?

Jeni   **Phone a Friend & Buddy Up**

When it comes to working out, if you can find a female friend to work out with, then all the better for you both. It's like having an accountability partner who can understand exactly what you're going through.

Sometimes women ask me why I don't suggest that they buddy up with their male other half, husband or boyfriend. Well, my reply to that is, his body is not going through the same changes that you are. He is unlikely to truly understand what a hot flash is, or how osteoporosis is affecting your bones, or the bladder weakness you are feeling when he keeps telling you that 'burpees & jumping jacks' are the only way to go with a full body workout! (It's not!).

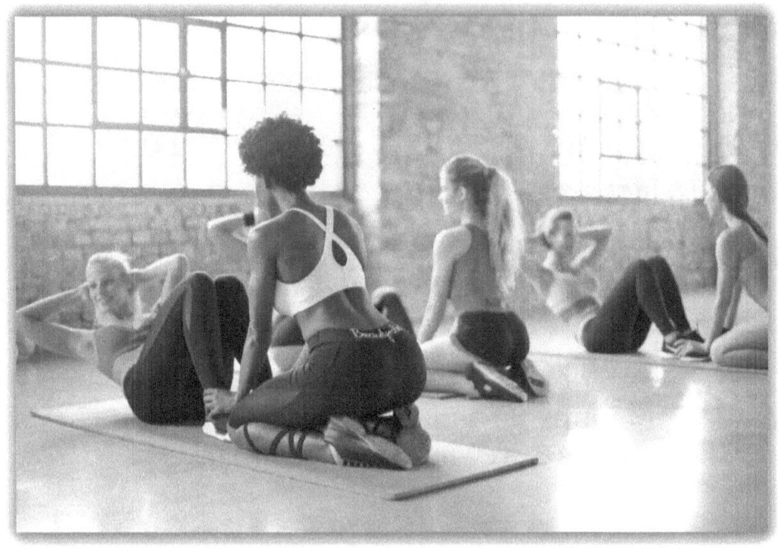

So, going for power walks, hitting the gym, cycling, swimming or attending a Zumba class with a mate will not only keep you accountable, it can help you lose weight faster, too.

Some researchers at the **Society of Behavioural Medicine** have found that friends who work out together are more likely to boost the calories they burn and can actually, help increase the duration of their active workouts.

The Biggest Challenges In Fitness & Weight Management Right Now

Domanique   So Jeni, Where are the big challenges in Fitness & weight management right now?

Jeni   **The Dairy and 'Lactose issue'**

Although some people make a conscious decision to actively stop eating & drinking dairy for their own personal reasons, there are a number of people who are either lactose intolerant or less commonly have an allergic reaction to lactose.

Intolerance means that the body is unable to digest the milk sugar 'lactose' which can cause any number of disagreeable side effects to your body including bloating, flatulence, diarrhoea, cramps & vomiting.

Whilst an **allergic reaction** to lactose, occurs when the body's immune system is triggered by drinking or eating dairy products; eg anaphylaxis

Domanique, did you know that the milk sugar lactose is broken down by the enzyme lactase in our body. Lactose intolerance is typically due to a low level of lactase in our gastrointestinal tract.

Now ladies, if you think you are lactose intolerant, it may be a good idea to keep a **food diary** of what you eat and when you are having digestive problems. If your digestive problems usually happen shortly after eating dairy, you may be lactose intolerant.

By the way, please don't believe that it can take 24 – 48 hours for your body to register lactose intolerance... That's a load of rubbish and actually applies to some cases of food poisoning, not food intolerances. If you are lactose intolerant, your intestines and bowels can let you know about it in as little as a few minutes or hours! Believe me!

Pre- & Pro-biotics are another important aspect of a good healthy gut. The fermentation process in some foods such has miso, yogurt, kimchi, and sauerkraut contain healthy bacteria. They give countless benefits that include preventing diarrhoea, bowel issues and strengthening the digestive system.

There are some excellent supplements that can also help, such has the **Arbonne Essentials Digestion Plus** that contains enzymes to help support the breakdown of lactose and I carry a couple of packets around with me everywhere I go. My husband won't let me leave the house without them, because he has seen how well they work.

Of course, some people also choose not to consume dairy due to the high fat content or because in some countries (illegal in the UK), dairy cows may have been given growth hormones.

As a farmer's wife, Domanique, I have had a real problem with digesting cow dairy well before I met my husband. My lactose intolerance could not cope with processing ice-cream, cheeses & butter etc.; this meant that I was not able to enjoy the labour of my husband toil! Ha-ha

Domanique   Ha-ha, so that's why you two got married, he was able to retain more of the profit, because you didn't drink it all. That's so funny!

Jeni   I know, right!

So, I have tried goats & soy milk, but I don't personally recommend either of these any more. I do however suggest dairy free / lactose free options such as; Rice, Almond, Hemp & Coconut milks

The Big Opportunities in Fitness & Weight Management Right Now

Domanique   This is great information, Jeni. So where are the big opportunities in fitness & weight management that many Professional women over 40 might be missing?

Jeni   **Get a coach** is an opportunity not to be missed Domanique.

Our lives are so busy and as we get older, we seem to acquire more and more responsibilities; home, partners, children, parents, job, business, pets etc. all impact on our time and so more professional women over 40 are struggling with being able to attend in-person weight management groups, fitness or gym sessions.

Fortunately, there are people like me who offer online social support that will encourage fitness & weight management every bit as much as in-person meetings.

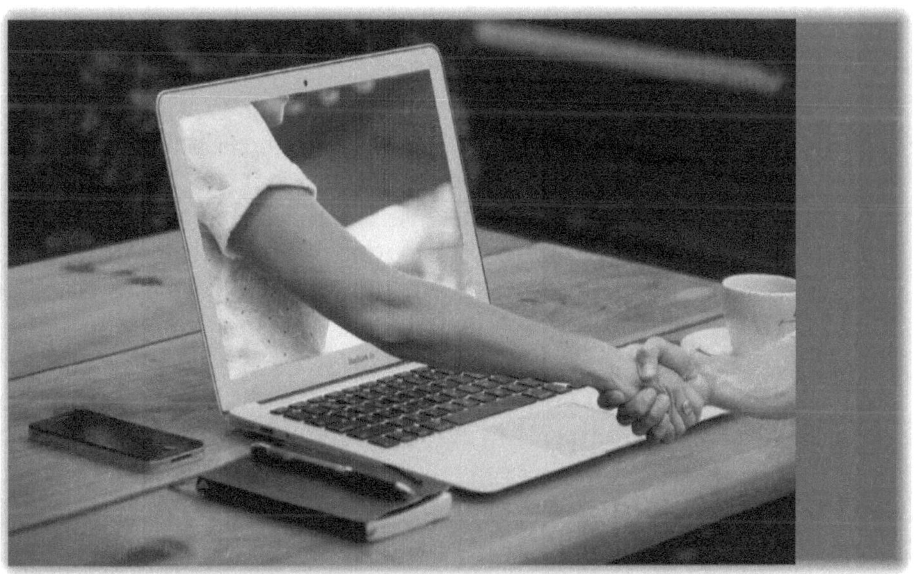

This kind of proactive support, professional guidance and weekly accountability can increase your chance of succeeding to reach your goal, help you stay focused, reactivate your physical energy levels, reformulate your healthy eating and assist you in the realisation that you can 'create the body you want to live in' so you can be Fit & Fab Forever!

Coaches are successful working with clients online and we are seeing amazing results, because we can be contacted and seen anywhere at any time. Even if factors such as mobility, dis-ability, child-care, elderly-parent care, work schedules, time zones etc. need to be taken into account.

Look at it this way Domanique, if your healthy eating and exercise are the ingredient you need to **'create the body you want to live in'**, then your Coach is the recipe book that will make sure that you use the ingredients in the right order and the correct amount to cook up the finished product you desire.

When you do seek out a Coach, it is important to note that they have agreed with you and covered:

- Full ParQ
- Goals – short & long term
- Weight & Measurements
- Current Eating habits
- Healthy Eating Schedule
- Allergies & Intolerances
- Sleep & Active Rest
- Religious & Cultural requirements
- Fitness & Exercise

Never go with a coach that only talks about fitness & exercise, without discussing what you eat, because that's only half the story!

How It's Easier To Get Started With The Ability To Manage Your Weight, Tone Your Body And Eat Better In 90 Days. Today

Domanique   Do you think it's easier or harder for a new Professional Woman Over 40 starting out today with Fitness & weight management than it was for you when you got started?

Jeni   I actually think it is so much easier for Professional Women over 40 to get started today with their fitness and weight management than ever before. This interview is full of tips, tricks & secrets that every woman can start TODAY. You don't need to wait to join a gym to start making a difference to your body.

Even a little bit of exercise can make a massive amount of difference! Being active really can help Professional women over 40 & especially those with menopausal symptoms. So if you exercise a little or a lot. I love the fact that research has shown that women who do some workout have fewer and milder daytime hot-flashes, night sweats and disturbed sleep.

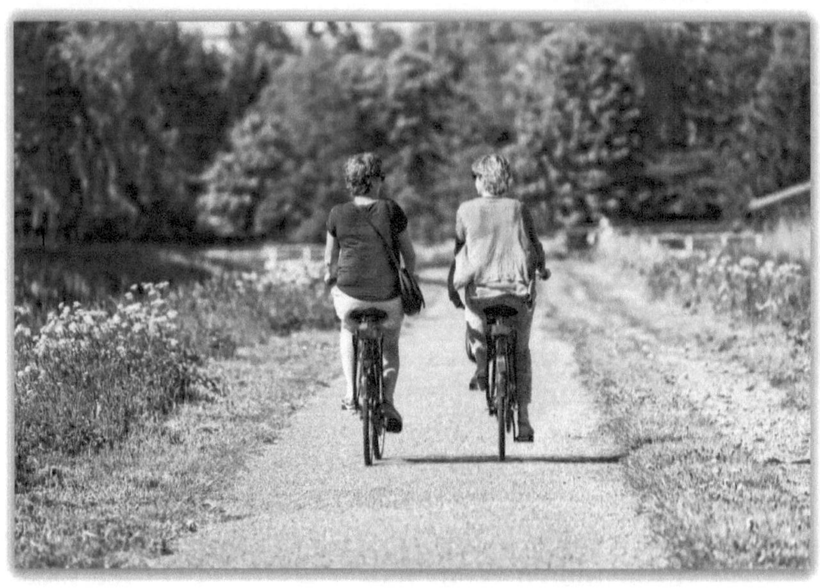

Menopausal low moods and even depression can be alleviated by the endorphins you create from exercising. Those 'feel-good chemicals' released during exercise can lift your mood and stave off anxiety.

I read Domanique that one of the latest studies, published by the **University of Applied Sciences in Tampere, Finland**, found that 49-year-old women who exercised regularly had a better quality of life and reduced menopausal symptoms.

The findings showed that those women who did exercise on a weekly basis from as little 1¼ hours jogging (15 mins x 5 days) or 2½ hours of fast walking (30 mins x 5 days), in addition to strength or balance training, such as yoga, HiiT or Pilates twice a week, were less likely to report anxiety, depression, problems with memory or concentration and even hot flushes.

Ladies, exercise will also help you control your weight at a time when hormones are conspiring against you to pile the fat around your middle. This is all the more important because being overweight can exacerbate menopausal symptoms.

Even More Fitness & Weight Management Tips, Tricks and Secrets

Domanique	Is there anything I haven't asked you about Fitness & weight management and the ability to manage your weight, tone your body and eat better in 90 days, that you'd like to share with our audience of Professional women over 40, Jeni?
Jeni	Yes, Domanique. I've shared a number of tips, tricks & a few secrets with you all today, but there are so many more I want to make sure you are aware of and I'm very quickly going to list these off for you as my **Top 10 count down:**

#10. Eat Your Carbs

Don't do yourself a disservice and cut out carbs completely. They matter! Eating carbs in the evening have been found to increase weight-loss and body-fat loss. Whilst consuming throughout the day can help you fight the bloating & sluggish digestion that regularly become an issue around the menopause.

#9. Breakfast like a King

We've all heard this saying and I know it's true. Have a heavy breakfast, full of goodness, it goes a long way in making you ready for the day and a light dinner is exactly what your body needs at the end of the day. A healthy breakfast can includes eggs, gluten free breads, oats, raisins, prunes, berries, fruits, spinach, fish, coconuts & avocados etc.

#8. Avoid processed foods & fast food

Please, please don't do it. Our bodies cannot process junk in the same way it did just a few years ago. They are high in saturated fat, which can slow down your digestion. In addition, most of these foods have little nutrition; they have been stripped of fibre, usually high in sugar & have very high fat content.

#7.   Eat a rich fibre diet

We need fibre for a healthy digestion system. Research shows that most Westerners get about half as much fibre as they need each day. Fibre adds bulk to stool, so it can move efficiently through the digestive system. Add more fibre slowly, because some vegetables and beans, can cause stomach discomfort and gas!

#6. Exercise to feel good, not "burn fat"

Over exercising and causing yourself an injury is never a good thing. Accidents happen, ligaments get torn and muscles get pulled; even multi-million pound footballers get benched due to muscle injuries. But you must take care to avoid over doing your exercises and burning out. After 40 years of age, it's great to exercise to feel good, not "burn fat". After all 'Burning fat' is a marketing term that doesn't mean anything!

#5. Cha cha Chia

I love Chia! With just 129 calories, less than 9g of fat alongside a massive 11g of fibre & 4 grams of protein per ounce, chia seeds can stabilise your blood sugar, boost weight loss, keep your hunger at bay and even help keep your body hydrated throughout the day.

#4 Don't drink your calories (unless it's an actual meal)

A major cause of weight gain is the consumption of calorie-filled or sugary drinks. Please stop drinking 'diet' 'low calorie' 'max' 'no added sugar' 'flavoured waters' & 'energy drinks'. 240 calories for a juice is wasted calories!

Check out the labels to see if 'no added sugar' actually means it's already full of sugar.

Did you know that sweeteners that add calories to a drink can go by many different names which are not always obvious to anyone looking at the ingredients list? Some common calorific sweeteners are listed below. If these appear in the ingredients list of your favourite refreshment, you are consumption a sugar-laden beverage.

- High-fructose corn syrup
- Fructose
- Fruit juice concentrates
- Honey
- Sugar
- Syrup
- Corn syrup
- Sucrose
- Dextrose

So ladies, ditch the sweetened drinks and consume water, decaffeinated coffee or tea, fresh mint or green teas instead.

#3   Eat a rainbow

Red & yellow & pink & green, purple & orange & blue! Well I don't know about blue, but you need to be eating as many colours as you can in the rainbow at every meal. The antioxidants, vitamins and minerals will work with your body and if you can eat raw, then all the better. 5-a-day is a good start!

#2   Get plenty of water

Whether you drink it or you eat it, women can get water through fruit, vegetables, soups, stews and more. If you are dehydrated, you can become constipated since your stool dries out in the digestive system and then you have a tough time expelling it. Like we don't have enough to deal with!

So although it might seem counterintuitive, drinking lots of water will also help reduce water-retention in the body. This is because a body that is dehydrated will try to hold on to the water it does have in preparation for the future. By telling your body that water is not in short supply, the fluid will be able to pass through unrestricted and do its job, such as flushing out the kidneys.

Drinking water before each meal also helps you feel fuller longer. It can help stop you over eating and snacking as much. You could also drink water in the form of homemade soup. Take it to work, have it as a starter; DON'T go for tinned soup if possible.

I always suggest that you have a glass of water beside the bed and if you like a slice of lemon seeping in it overnight, all the better. By drinking water first thing in the morning, you are setting your gut up for a great day! Because, after 8 hours sleep (well hopefully 8 hours sleep), our body becomes dehydrated. So water will:

- Increase the flow of oxygen & help our blood cells & muscles
- Boost our metabolism by about 24% which can assist in maintaining a healthy weight.
- It helps to clean your colon, so nutrients can be more easily absorbed.
- The brain tissue is 76% water & needs hydration so you don't feel tired, have headaches or experience major mood swings

#1   It's all in the mind!

Decide to do it and stick to it! Will power is key! Be accountable! However, you want to put it, you must make the decision to achieve your fitness & weight management and have a positive outlook in life and think about your fitness level to help you support your family and friends when they need you.

Nothing I say or do will help you, if you're not ready to make any of these changes and suggestion real. Only YOU can decide and realise that it is possible.

You have to make the decision to **'create the body you want to live in'.**

More About The Ability To Manage Your Weight, Tone Your Body And Eat Better In 90 Days and Jeni Bennett

Domanique   Jeni, How can people find out more about you and what you do?

Jeni   Well, Domanique, they can find out more about me and what I am doing in so many ways. I have my Fit & Fab Forever course & training:

- Online mini workshops
- Teleseminars
- Zoom Webinars
- Live Workshops in libraries, community & non-profit events
- Private Intensive 1:1 sessions
- Private VIP ½ Intensive Day
- Private VIP Day
- 30 Day Challenge Coaching Packages
- 30 Days to Healthy Living & Beyond
- Fit & Fab Forever 90 Day Course + Private Coaching Program
- Fit & Fab Forever 90 Day Course + VIP Intensive Day Coaching Package
- Speaking events

- Freelance Consulting
- Twice Yearly Retreat - One is in the UK and One is in Europe or the Rest of the World.

So if any of you Professional ladies over 40 are seeking a Coach or Mentor that understands your personal needs, as well as how you can

'Create the body you want to live in'

You can find me over at www.jenibennett.com

Or Email me for further details at
Jeni@jenibennett.com

However ladies, please note that this may not be for you if:

- What you are already doing is working for you
- You wake up with loads of energy
- You love the gym and can easily spend a couple of hours a day there
- You are in the best shape ever in your life
- You don't believe you can do any of this!

Finally

Domanique: Well thank you Jeni Bennett for a great interview. I'm sure all the professional women over 40 in our audience have gotten a ton of value from tips, tricks and secrets about fitness & weight management that you shared. This was some real insider stuff. Thank you very much for sharing with us so graciously. It's been great and thank you all the professional women over 40 in our audience for joining us for this amazing presentation about tips, tricks and tools with fitness & weight management that can help you massively improve your results.

Have a great day.

Jeni Bennett: Thank you, Domanique for the interview. I really appreciate it.

References

National Institutes of Health. (2015). Stress urinary incontinence. Retrieved May 13, 2016, from https://www.nlm.nih.gov/medlineplus/ency/article/000891.htm

Office on Women's Health. (2012). Urinary incontinence fact sheet. Retrieved May 13, 2016, from http://www.womenshealth.gov/publications/our-publications/fact-sheet/urinary-incontinence.html

http://www.dailymail.co.uk/health/article-2997794/What-menopause-REALLY-does-body-tell-started-continuing-ultimate-guide-surviving-change.html

Goodwin, J. (2012). What Causes Hot Flashes, Anyway? Retrieved April 27, 2016, from http://consumer.healthday.com/women-s-health-information-34/estrogen-news-238/what-causes-hot-flashes-anyway-663671.html

Heitkemper, M.M. & Chang, L. (2009). Do Fluctuations in Ovarian Hormones Affect Gastrointestinal Symptoms in Women With Irritable Bowel Syndrome? Gender Medicine, 6(Suppl 2), 152-167. doi: 10.1016/j.genm.2009.03.004 https://www.34-menopause-symptoms.com/digestive-problems/articles/

Dr Kristina Routh, Freelance Health Editor, Bupa Health Content Team, February 2018

Miss Shirin Irani, Consultant Gynaecologist

Lisa Jubilee - http://www.lisajubileenutrition.com/

Tena –
https://www.tena.co.uk/tenalady/about-incontinence/causes-of-female-incontinence/

Lisiana Carter -
https://www.consumerhealthdigest.com/menopause-center/

https://www.eatthis.com

https://www.quora.com/What-percentage-of-new-gym-members-in-January-stop-coming-after-February

University of Applied Sciences in Tampere, Finland

Dr. Michael Forman Miami clinical nutritionist

Jennifer Keirstead – Nutritionist

Lauren Slayton, MS, RD, and founder of Foodtrainers.

Johns Hopkins Bloomberg School of Public Health.

www.ingramcontent.com/pod-product-compliance
Lightning Source LLC
Chambersburg PA
CBHW031418250726
48656CB00002B/718